Through **meditation**
we reach out towards the
ideal

Contents
page

Understanding
the processes

that shape and create our inner and outer world forms part of the pathway to wisdom. The vast range of meditative traditions agree that it is understanding that frees us.

(Christina Feldman)

Introduction

There are many reasons why people begin and continue the practice of relaxation and meditation. Although traditionally meditation was practiced for spiritual purposes, today there are many other reasons and benefits associated with regular practice. Relaxation and meditation can assist in reducing stress and anxiety; improving health and well-being; feeling more relaxed and peaceful; coping better with everyday life and its challenges; and increasing self-awareness.

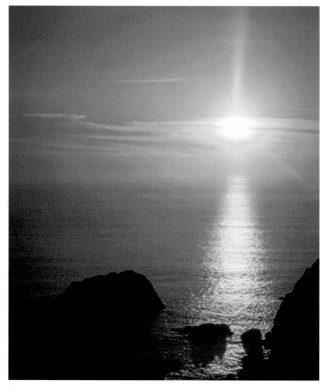

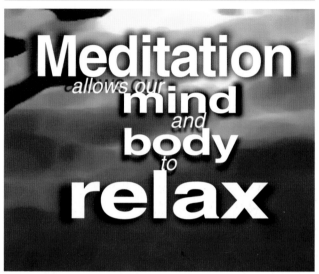

Meditation allows our mind and body to relax. When meditating we let go of the pressures, anxieties and constant 'doing' of our everyday life. It is a natural, healthy way to reduce our stress levels. Furthermore, the benefits of meditation are lasting - increasing our feelings of inner peace and our ability to cope better with the challenges that we all experience. People who meditate regularly experience increased energy, vitality, efficiency and confidence in their everyday life.

Meditation is a pathway to health and well-being. When we meditate our body's natural state of balance is restored. When our body is out of balance our immune system is compromised. Whereas when our body is in a state of balance its natural healing and repairing abilities are at their

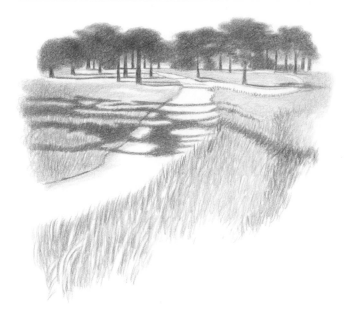

best. The result is improved health, more energy and vitality and a general feeling of well-being.

Meditation is also a pathway to greater self-awareness. A process in which we gradually come to know and understand ourselves more fully. As we become more in tune with ourselves, creativity is re-awakened and we discover our talents and realise the unlimited potential we each have. Intuition and imagination, which are re-discovered through meditation, are essential ingredients for creativity. Focusing within, we start to appreciate our true nature. Regular meditation can lead to greater self-acceptance, self-worth and self-love. It can also lead to greater empathy, understanding and love of others.

Meditation does not have to involve the acceptance of any particular religious or philosophical beliefs, nor is it an escape from reality. Rather it is a process through which we gain insight and clarity into our own true nature and the nature of reality. This inner wisdom provides us with the skills and tools to deal more effectively with the challenges our lives may bring.

With regular meditation we can experience a profound inner peace. We may find that a sense of joy, gratitude and love for life is re-awakened, and consequently we see life as something exciting and wonderful.

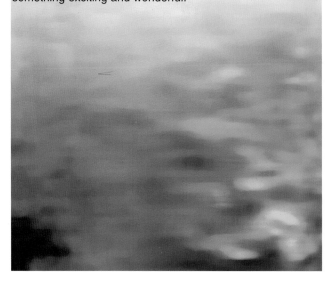

What is Meditation?

Meditation is a timeless, natural process in which we quieten our mind and experience our own true nature. When we are not 'doing' anything, and there are no distractions we are left with our essence.

Taking the time to quieten our mind and enter the stillness, we relax, and the 'doing' stops. In our everyday lives our minds are generally focused outwards. We are preoccupied with our outer world - other people; the things we have to do; things which have happened in the past; concerns about the future, and so on. When we meditate, we focus our attention inwards, and experience 'being' rather than 'doing'. In this stillness, we experience the 'now' moment which is free from the pressures and stresses of everyday life - from our doubts and fears. **Whereas 'doing' is a state of focused, directed, goal-oriented activity, 'being' is a state where we fully experience the present moment.** 'Being' and 'doing' are equally important and need equal attention if we are to feel whole and balanced. The 'being' state, however, allows us to replenish and revitalise ourselves.

'Meditation' refers more to a state of mind, than to an activity. **We have all experienced the inner stillness of meditation, whether we are aware of it or not.** For example, daydreaming is a form of meditation - when we are lost in the beauty of a sunset; mesmerised by the rhythm of the sea; or when we just stop to experience the sun's warmth upon our shoulders.

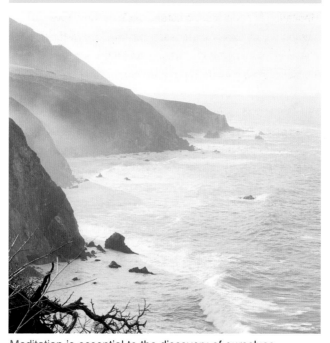

Meditation is essential to the discovery of ourselves. Although understanding oneself is of primary importance, many of us avoid forming a relationship with our true self by making ourselves busy. When we sit in meditation we learn communication with our true self, and get in touch with our inner life of feelings. Meditation enables us to discover our talents, our wisdom, our creative ability and our unlimited potential. In meditation we learn to go beyond the limitations of the logical mind with its linear thoughts and rational beliefs, into the inspirational and intuitive. **The true self cannot be grasped by logical thinking alone.**

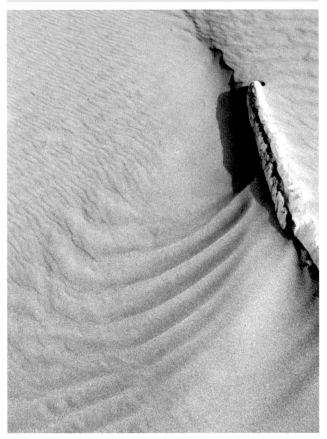

The profound inner peace we experience as a result of meditation brings with it greater understanding, empathy, clarity, compassion and acceptance of ourselves and others. It Enables us to meet the challenges of life with a far more balanced and harmonious attitude.

What Happens When We Meditate?

When we are meditating we experience an altered state of consciousness in which our mind is relaxed, but very alert. It is the nature of our mind to be constantly busy with thoughts. Only when these thoughts and the busyness of our minds are quietened can we see with clarity.

When we meditate our mind, body and spirit is in a state of balance and harmony. We become intimate with our inner life, inner wisdom, intuition.

Many things happen to our physiology during this process - the rhythm of our brain-waves slow down; our heart-beat slows; our respiration rate decreases and our blood pressure drops. All these things are healthy and necessary for balance and harmony in mind and body.

The opposite applies when we are feeling stressed, frustrated or angry - the rhythm of our brain-waves speed up; our heart rate increases; breath becomes shallow and rapid; and blood pressure rises.

Meditation is a very powerful remedy for stress relief.

How Can Meditation Relieve Stress?

Excessive stress is a common cause of illness and disease. When we are stressed our body becomes out of balance and our immune system is weakened, as is our resistance to dis-ease. (Disease in the body being a state of dis-ease in our mind and emotions.)

Stress in itself is not bad. We all need a little stress to motivate and excite us. However, too much stress can push us beyond our capacity to cope.

Many of the challenges we meet in everyday life can hold the potential for stress and tension - things such as deadlines; work demands; lack of work; finances; ambition; insufficient time for ourselves; fear of the future; relationships; competitiveness; and even our level of self-awareness can create stress.

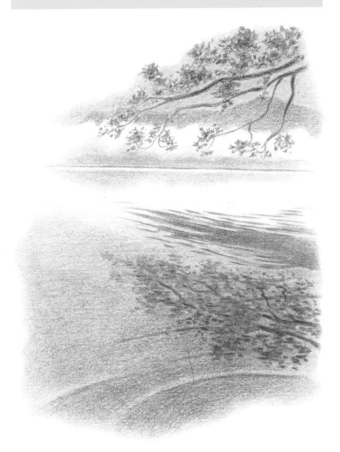

We become stressed when our 'Fight or Flight' response is activated. This is our bodies normal, automatic response to fearful or challenging situations. Our body prepares to 'fight the enemy' or 'run for its life'.

Meditation

The way our body prepares for this is by tensing muscles; elevating our heart rate; elevating our blood pressure; and

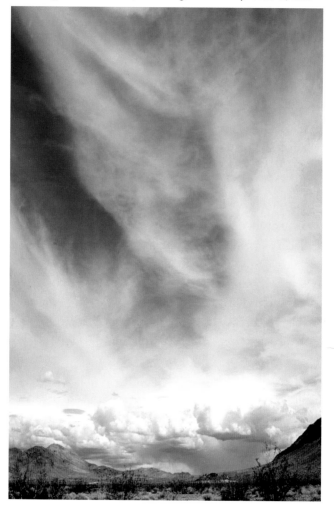

secreting adrenaline and hormones. In this state, our body is now prepared to either 'fight' or 'run'. After the intense activity of fighting or running, our body chemistry then returns to normal.

However most of the fearful or challenging situations we encounter in our lives today do not require us to fight or run. In our complex and competitive society, we are faced with many emotional and mental stressors - fears about the future; dealing with people who annoy us; meeting deadlines; confrontations etc. Similarly, we experience stress when we have issues that we have repressed or chosen not to confront - old memories; hurt; guilt; anger; resentment and grief. Our muscles become primed for 'Fight or Flight' but do not have an appropriate outlet. With no outlet - no intense activity - there is no tension release, and so our stress levels continue to build. Too much stress causes an imbalance within our body and within our natural healing processes. Symptoms such as headache, fatigue, inability to concentrate and insomnia are very often stress related.

Stress does not only affect the body. Our state of mind is also affected. When we are stressed we can become intolerant, irritable and impatient. We are much more likely to have negative attitudes and our level of concentration can be impaired. In this state of mind we tend to overreact and not cope as well with life's challenges.

Meditation

Although we cannot control all the challenges we encounter, we can control our attitude and the way we respond. When we cultivate inner calmness, understanding and compassion through the practice of meditation, we view our challenges with clarity, and are able to move through them with courage and optimism. The habitual nature of our reactions can be transformed through meditation and self-awareness.

When we meditate our mind and body relax and our body chemistry returns to normal. This state of inner peace is also carried over into our everyday lives, empowering and enabling us to make more balanced and harmonious choices.

**Through meditation,
we learn skills to stay centred
and peaceful in the midst
of the stressful and challenging
situations we all experience.
Meditation provides us with
the inner resources to approach
these situations with greater
understanding and compassion.**

The Practice of Meditation

Breathing:
Breathing is an important aspect of relaxation and meditation.

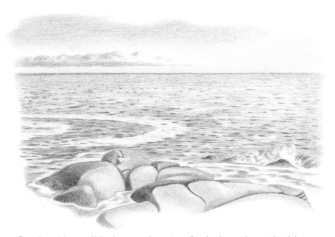

Our health, well-being and state of mind are inextricably linked with the way we breathe. When stressed, our breathing is shallow and rapid. We can learn to control the way we feel by controlling our breathing. Deliberate, deep, slow breaths bring about a state of relaxation.

There are many breathing techniques for meditation, one is to breathe in through the nose - completely filling the abdomen with air - and then completing each cycle by exhaling through the mouth. **Refer pages 26 and 27 for relaxation exercise.**

Once a state of relaxation has been reached, we can allow our breathing to take on its own rhythm.

Meditation

Posture and Position

Some cultures and traditions emphasise sitting cross-legged in the lotus position for meditation. This is an ideal position for our posture and energy flow, but not essential and can be rather difficult and uncomfortable for those who do not regularly sit this way.

An ideal posture, but not essential.

The most important consideration is our comfort. We cannot become relaxed if our body is uncomfortable. It is desirable our backs are straight to assist the free flow of blood and energy.

Lying on our back with arms and legs uncrossed is a good position, as is sitting in a comfortable chair with our hands placed palms-up in our laps and our feet placed flat on the floor.

Creating A Special Place:

It is helpful to have a special place where we go to meditate - a certain chair; corner of the room etc. When we go to a customary place, particularly in early stages of our meditation practice, we begin to associate this with relaxation and thoughts of peace, so assisting in the relaxation process.

It is also helpful if we feel that this special place is one of beauty and peace. It should feel like a retreat from the 'doing' of everyday life. To enhance this feeling, it assists if we surround our special place with items that reflect beauty and peace - flowers, crystals - whatever items symbolise beauty, peace and love.

Tranquil music playing in the background may aid the relaxation process, as can tapes of peaceful sounds such as running water, thunderstorms etc. Anything can be used which has a soothing effect. Aromatherapy may assist. Many essential oils reduce stress and promote relaxation, such as Lavender, Clary Sage and Geranium.

We also help create a relaxing atmosphere by surrounding our special place with colours which we feel have a nurturing or calming effect, particularly pastel colours. Bright colours such as red may be enlivening, but not conducive to relaxation. Just as you have surrounded your special place with items reflecting beauty and peace, surround it with colours that reflect relaxation - perhaps wear certain coloured clothes, or have special cushions. Be creative - this is your special place.

Ensure the light in your special place isn't too bright, and you are both warm and comfortable.

Your special place should be pleasing and nurturing to your senses.

When To Meditate

Many traditions advocate meditating at sunrise and sunset. Early morning certainly has its advantages because it is the time when our mind is the clearest and least cluttered. Some find meditating in the morning prepares them for the day ahead. Others find meditating in the evening beneficial for releasing the stresses of the day and assisting a good night's sleep.

Try to meditate at a time that fits in with your routine—a time when you know you are not going to be interrupted.

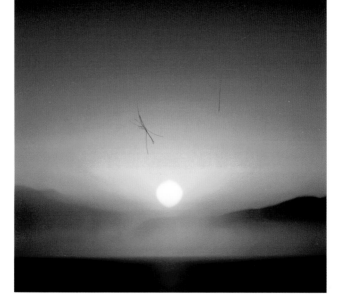

How Long Should Each Meditation Be?

When starting a meditation practice, it is best to gradually increase the length of each meditation. Start with 10 minutes and build to 30 minutes per meditation.

If you have limited time, it may be useful to set an alarm to mark the end of your meditation. However, ensure that it is distant or muffled so as not to startle you .

Because of our varied lifestyles and routines, it is necessary for each of us to find a time of day and length of time that best suits our needs. It is more beneficial to meditate for 15 minutes than not at all.

Ensure you don't make meditation into a chore that must be done - sitting there wondering when time is up. It is a time for 'being' and surrendering to the experience. It should be enjoyable and nurturing. It is a special time for getting to know yourself.

The Challenge Of A Busy Mind

The biggest challenge people experience when meditating is a busy mind or lapses of attention. This is an entirely normal experience for all of us.

It is the nature of our mind to have thoughts, images and memories. Meditation does not endeavour to push these thoughts away. Rather, the aim is to develop the ability to let thoughts and images 'float' by without being drawn into them. Simply accept and acknowledge these thoughts or images and then gently bring your attention back to the focus of your meditation.

When we resist our thoughts or become impatient with ourselves we hinder the meditation process. Becoming impatient or questioning what we are experiencing, or wondering what we 'should' be experiencing, are also distractions which engage our logical mind, to the detriment of the meditative state.

With a little practice we learn how to 'flow' with distractions, rather than question or judge our experience.

How To Finish Meditation:
Once we have finished our meditation, it is best to return to normal waking consciousness very gently and slowly - taking a few minutes to feel the effects of the meditation.

When feeling ready gently stretch the limbs, open eyes and return to normal waking consciousness.

Relaxation

The process of relaxation is a prerequisite to deeper states of meditation. When we are in a relaxed state our body has a chance to regain its natural balance. When our body is in a state of balance it maintains, replenishes and heals itself.

The fundamental relaxation technique involves correct posture, deep breathing and consciously relaxing our body parts one by one.

Meditation begins once we are in a relaxed state.

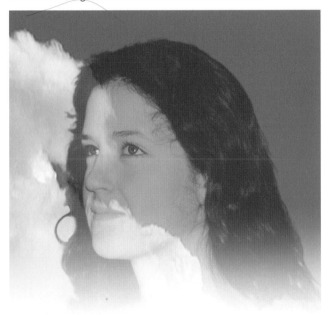

Relaxation Exercise

Select your relaxation position. For the purpose of this and the following exercises let us assume you are seated in a chair. Get comfortable, and ensure arms and legs are uncrossed and your back is straight (loosen any tight clothing, belts, shoes etc). When you feel comfortable, close you eyes and begin focusing your attention on a comfortable breathing pattern. Then begin taking deep, full breaths. As you breathe in through your nose feel your abdomen expand. As you breathe out through your mouth feel your abdomen contract. Spend a few minutes consciously breathing deeply. Then allow yourself to breathe naturally.

- Focus your attention on your right foot - clench it - then allow it to relax completely and fully.

- Place your attention on your left foot - clench it - then allow it to relax completely and fully.

- Focus on your right leg - clench the muscles in your leg - and then let them relax.

- Focus on your left leg - clench the muscles in your leg - and then let them relax. Feel your thigh muscles in both legs letting go and becoming limp and loose.

- Place your attention on your buttocks - clench your buttocks - and then release the tension.

- Focus on your back - your beautiful strong back muscles - upper, middle and lower. Tense your back muscles - experience what tension feels like - and then let go completely, feeling all tension drain.

Imagine your stomach and chest muscles - tighten these muscles and feel the tension - then let go completely.

Place your awareness in your right arm - tighten the muscles in your right arm - and then let them go - let them relax.

Place your awareness in your left arm - tighten the muscles in your left arm - and then let them go - let them relax.

Next concentrate on your neck - tense the muscles in your neck and shoulders - and just let go - let all tension drain way.

Place your attention on your face - tighten your jaw muscles, and the muscles around your eyes - and then release the tension - feel your jaw drop open slightly, the muscles around your eyes relax and your forehead become smooth and free of tension.

If there are any areas of tension left in your body, place your concentration in those areas and imagine them relaxing and letting go - all tension draining away.

Spend a few minutes in this relaxed state, feeling the peace and tranquillity - the inner stillness.

A variation on the above relaxation, is to go through each of your body parts (as above), however instead of tensing and then relaxing them, simply imagine each of your body parts relaxing, and how this feels.

Observation/Mindfulness Meditation

**Meditation generally falls into two categories:
Observation Or Concentration.**

Observation Meditation is passive. During this process we notice our inner thoughts and feelings, but do not react to them or join in with them. We also notice external distractions and sounds, but once again do not react. Rather, we observe everything happening within and without us, allowing it to float by without judgment. We are not to engage our logical mind by wondering whether a thought or image is relevant or not; nor should we question whether the meditation is going well. The purpose of observation meditation is to let go of our logical mind, and just allow ourselves to be in the 'now' moment.

Within this state we are able to notice what is taking place beneath our logical minds - beneath our thoughts, beliefs and attitudes. Being in the now moment can bring clarity, understanding and insight.

We have the opportunity of seeing things how they really are, by moving beyond our thoughts, beliefs, judgments and attitudes, all of which colour our world.

Though Observation Meditation we can begin to understand our true nature. It is a pathway to self-discovery and self-awareness. We also have the opportunity to begin to understand the true nature of all things - the universal principles which apply to all things. Observation meditation can lead to an understanding of reality, which is far more expanded than the reality defined by our logical mind and coloured by our beliefs, judgements and attitudes.

Observation Exercise

Seated in a chair, get comfortable, and ensure arms and legs are uncrossed and the back is straight (loosen any tight clothing, belts, shoes etc). When you feel comfortable, close your eyes and begin focusing attention on a comfortable breathing pattern. Then begin taking deep, full breaths. As you breathe in through your nose feel your abdomen expand. As you breathe out through your mouth feel your abdomen contract. Spend two or three minutes consciously breathing deeply. Then let go and allow yourself to breathe naturally. (If you need to relax more fully, go through the 'relaxation' exercise before commencing your observation meditation).

You may use your breath as a focus to keep you anchored in the 'now' moment, however do not focus on the breath to the exclusion of everything else. Notice any thoughts or images - acknowledge them, and let them float by. Do not question or judge them - just allow them to be. Notice any outer noises or distractions - acknowledge them and allow them to go. Do not judge them as 'right' or 'wrong'. Just allow yourself to 'be' and allow whatever comes.

Attempt to spend at least 15 minutes in this observation meditation, and then when you feel ready, gently bring yourself back to normal waking consciousness. Make a note in a journal of any insights or experiences you might have had.

Concentration Meditation

The object of concentration meditation is to become focused on one thing to the exclusion of everything else.

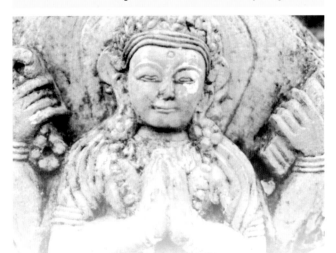

There are many things we can choose to concentrate on. We can choose to focus on our breath - on the natural rhythm of our breath as it rises and falls. We may choose to focus on a mantra - a sound which can be chanted as a form of meditation. Sound can be powerful, transforming and healing. The Sanskrit word 'OM' is said to be the sound from which the universe arises, and is often used in the practice of meditation. However, we may choose a word that has meaning for us such as 'love', 'peace', 'relax' etc. and repeat it over and over during our meditation.

A further option, is choosing to concentrate on objects - particularly those which invoke powerful feelings of love, peace and beauty. Objects which are often used as the focus of observation in meditation are crystals; flowers; the flame of a candle; or symbols of the Divine Being, Enlightened Beings or Oneness - such as God, Christ, Allah, Buddha, Brahman, etc.

If there is a preference to meditate out of doors, then we may use the beauty of nature for concentration meditation - perhaps a beautiful sunset; white fluffy clouds; the peaceful sound of bird songs; the sound of a babbling brook; the rhythm of the sea; or the feeling and sound of the breeze as it caresses us.

Another technique is to concentrate on a feeling or quality - perhaps something that we would like more of in our lives. We can choose such things as 'love' - focusing on the feeling of being surrounded by love, filled with love and emanating love. Or perhaps we might choose 'peace' - focusing on the feeling of being peaceful, having inner peace, being balanced and harmonious.

Concentration meditation can lead us to merge with and experience the essence of the object of our focus, bringing with it expanded awareness and insight.

The practice of concentration meditation enables us to experience the 'now' moment, free from our logical mind with its thoughts, beliefs, judgments and attitudes. It is a freeing and empowering experience.

Concentration Exercise

1. Seated in a chair, get comfortable, and ensure your arms and legs are uncrossed and your back is straight (loosen any tight clothing, belts, shoes etc). When you feel comfortable, close your eyes and begin focusing your attention on a comfortable breathing pattern. Then begin taking deep, full breaths. As you breathe in through your nose feel your abdomen expand. As you breathe out through your mouth feel your abdomen contract. Spend two to three minutes consciously breathing deeply. Then, let go and allow yourself to breathe naturally. If you need to relax more fully, go through the 'relaxation' exercise previously described, before commencing your concentration meditation.

   Breathing naturally, focus your attention on your breath as you inhale and exhale. Feel the cooling intake and the warmer exhalation. Notice the movement and feeling of your body with each breath. Become one with your breath.

   Attempt to spend at least 15 minutes in this concentration meditation, and then when you feel ready, gently bring yourself back to normal waking consciousness. Make a note in a journal of any insights or experiences you may have had.

2. Select an object on which to concentrate (in this instance, let us say a flower, but it can be any object). Seated in a chair, get comfortable, and ensure your arms and legs

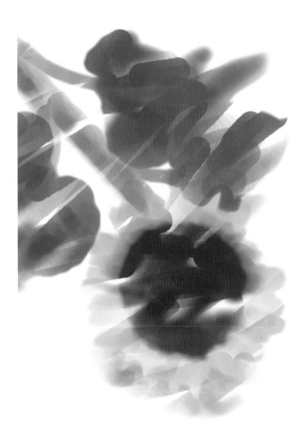

are uncrossed and your back is straight (loosen any tight clothing, belts, shoes etc).

Meditation

When you feel comfortable, close your eyes and begin focusing your attention on your natural breath. Then begin taking deep, full breaths. As you breathe in through your nose feel your abdomen expand. As you breathe out through your mouth feel your abdomen contract. Spend a few minutes consciously breathing deeply. Then let go and allow yourself to breathe naturally. If you need to relax more fully, go through the 'relaxation' exercise previously described, before commencing your concentration meditation.

Then breathing naturally and in your own rhythm, open your eyes and focus your attention on the flower (object) that you have selected. Become one with the flower. Feel yourself as the flower. See everything there is to see about the flower. Use your other senses if you wish - what does the flower smell like? What does it feel like? Imagine what it would sound like if you could hear it. Imagine yourself as the flower - what is its experience of life.

Attempt to spend at least 15 minutes in this concentration meditation, and then when you feel ready, gently bring yourself back to normal waking consciousness. Make a note in a journal of any insights or experiences you may have had .

3. Select a mantra or a word, such as 'OM', 'love', 'peace' - whatever has meaning for you. Seated in a chair, get comfortable, and ensure your arms and legs are uncrossed and your back is straight (loosen any tight clothing, belts, shoes etc). When you feel comfortable, close your eyes and begin focusing attention on a comfortable breathing pattern. Then begin taking deep, full breaths. As you breathe in through your nose feel your abdomen expand. Breathing out through your mouth feel your abdomen contract. Spend a few minutes consciously breathing deeply. Then let go and allow yourself to breathe naturally. If you need to relax more fully, go through the 'relaxation' exercise previously described, before commencing your concentration meditation.

Focus your attention on your natural breath and with every exhalation repeat your mantra out loud. Feel yourself resonate with the sound of the word and become one with it. Remain focused on your mantra and the resonance and feelings that you experience. Become absorbed into the sound.

Attempt to spend at least 15 minutes in this concentration meditation, and then when you feel ready, gently bring yourself back to normal waking consciousness. Make a note in a journal of any insights or experiences you may have had.

Inner Wisdom Meditation

In a meditative state, when our thoughts, beliefs, judgments and perceptions are silenced, we are able to get in touch with our inner wisdom - our inner knowing and intuition.

We may focus our attention upon specific subjects, questions or issues. In this state of expanded awareness when all thoughts and concerns are quietened, we are able to see with clarity and wisdom. We may choose to pose questions about everyday challenges: "Should I take the job?" "What are my true feelings about this issue?"

If we want insight into why we are in a state of ill health or dis-ease, we can ask questions such as: "What is causing this illness within me?" "How may I help myself heal?"

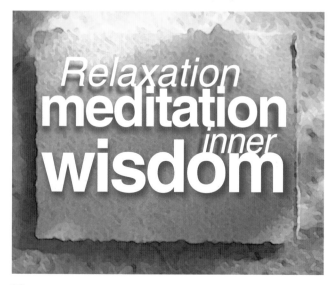

We can also use our inner wisdom as a general guide throughout life, posing questions such as: "Is there anything I need to know right now?", "What aspects of my life need attention?"

In the same way, the mysteries of life and the universe may be meditated upon, posing question such as: "Who am I?", "What is my purpose in life?", "Who or what is God?" etc.

Inner Wisdom Meditation is a powerful tool for uncovering true feelings, gaining insight and clarity into our personality, habits and motivations.

After posing a question, we may receive information or images whilst still in a meditative state, or answers may come to us when we are going about our everyday life. Sometimes answers come in very unexpected forms, so it is of benefit to remain open - without either expectations or judgement. An answer may come through a feeling, a vision, a dream, or we may just 'know' instinctively. The issue or question is not necessarily focused upon in meditation (our logical mind is not engaged). Rather, we go into meditation with an intention, and our subconscious mind works on our answer, free from the interference of our conscious mind. The answer may come straight away, overnight, or it may take several days. Be patient and persevere.

Inner Wisdom Exercise

Select an issue, question or challenge for which you would like an answer or clarity. Get clear on your question and then let it go, knowing that your subconscious mind knows what your intention is. Seated in a chair, get comfortable, and ensure arms and legs are uncrossed and your back is straight (loosen any tight clothing, belts, shoes etc). When you feel comfortable, close your eyes and begin focusing attention on your natural breath. Then begin taking deep, full breaths. As you breathe in through your nose feel your abdomen expand. As you breathe out through your mouth, feel your abdomen contract. Spend a few minutes consciously breathing deeply. Then let go and allow yourself to breathe naturally. If you need to relax more fully, go through the 'relaxation' exercise previously described, before commencing your inner wisdom meditation.

Then breathing naturally, go into a state of observation meditation. Notice any thoughts, feelings or images that occur, but do not react to them (refer to 'Observation Meditation' previously described).

Attempt to spend at least 15 minutes in meditation. When you feel ready, gently return to waking consciousness. Write in a journal any insights or experiences you may have had . If you do not have any immediate answers or insights, remain open - your answers can come in unexpected forms, such as in something you read, or something you watch on TV, or in conversation with someone.

Dynamic Meditation - Visualisation

Unlike Observation Meditation which is passive, visualisation is dynamic - we direct the thoughts and images of our mind. The uses of visualisation are unlimited.

In its simplest form, we can use visualisation for stress relief - imagining ourselves in a beautiful, peaceful place in nature. Perhaps walking through a tropical rainforest alive with wildlife; or along a deserted beach feeling at peace and at one with the rhythm of the waves; diving with whales and dolphins; floating on fluffy white clouds; soaring as an eagle high above the earth - whatever holds beauty, wonder and peace for us. Just as with Concentration Meditation we choose a focus for our attention, however when visualising, our images provide the focus for our attention.

A further use of visualisation is to imagine the life we want and to manifest those things we would like to have accompany us through our life. We can create anything that we can imagine. We are constantly imagining whether we are aware of it or not. When we worry about something or have a negative thought about ourselves, we visualise it and it is imprinted upon our subconscious mind. When our subconscious mind gets a 'picture' it tends to create this image in reality. We can choose to consciously create thoughts and images of health, abundance, prosperity and well-being.

We may want to create a fulfilling job; a loving, nurturing relationship; perfect health; peace and happiness - abundance and prosperity in all its forms. Or we may want to improve our self-worth and self-love by changing a limiting or core belief we may have about ourselves. In this instance, we may imagine ourselves as confident rather than 'shy'; loved rather than 'unloved'; intelligent rather than 'stupid'; successful rather than a 'failure'; or enthusiastic and passionate about life rather than 'bored and disinterested'.

Visualisation can be used as a powerful tool for achieving our goals - imagining ourselves at our ideal weight; visualising ourselves whole and healthy in mind, body and spirit; seeing ourselves successfully completing our goals; visualising ourselves in a nurturing, loving, happy relationship; imagining ourselves as having a fulfilling and rewarding job, etc.

Using all of our senses makes visualisation much more powerful and real within our subconscious. When we include our senses - sight, smell, taste, touch and hearing - it makes our image come alive.

So too are our visualisations still more powerful by bringing strong emotions and feeling to them. We can experience such things as joy at having achieved our goal, happiness at having manifested our desire; courage and strength at having overcome perceived limitations; optimism about the future; enthusiasm and love for life; and energy and vitality. The more powerful the image, the more strongly it will imprint itself upon our subconscious mind.

Visualisations and affirmations are powerful tools for creating the reality we want.

Visualisation Exercise

Inner Sanctuary

Seated in a chair, get comfortable, and ensure arms and legs are uncrossed and the back is straight (loosen any tight clothing, belts, shoes etc). When you feel comfortable, close your eyes and begin focusing your attention on a comfortable breathing pattern. Then begin taking deep, full breaths. As you breathe in through your nose feel your abdomen expand. As you breathe out through your mouth feel your abdomen contract. Spend a few minutes consciously breathing deeply. Let go and allow yourself to breathe naturally. If you need to relax more fully, go through the 'relaxation' exercise before commencing your visualisation.

In your imagination, you are going to create an Inner Sanctuary - this will be your own special place where you

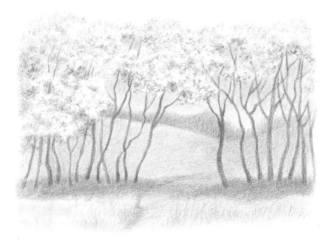

can go to feel at peace, for healing, for balance - a retreat where you feel safe, loved, peaceful and nurtured.

Use your imagination to visualise where you would like your inner sanctuary to be - perhaps on a sunlit beach; in a beautiful rainforest; beside a river draped with willow - wherever is beautiful to you. Imagine this scene as completely as possible. What is the weather like? - feel the sun upon your shoulders, or the cold wind upon your face. Can you smell anything? - flowers, trees, dampness, fresh air? Can you hear anything? - birds, insects, running water? Spend some time exploring your special place - use your senses.

Now imagine a structure in this special place. It may be a building, a temple, a cave, a tree house - it may be very elaborate or very simple. Just allow whatever comes to you without judgement. You may build it yourself if you wish, or you may see it already existing. Spend some time exploring and discovering this special structure. You may wish to paint or decorate it.

Now enter your structure - your sanctuary. Notice what is in your sanctuary and notice what is not in your sanctuary. How does it look? How does it feel? How does it smell? Spend a little time exploring and discovering the inside of your sanctuary.

When your visualisation is complete, gently bring yourself back to waking consciousness.

Achieving Goals:

Select a goal you would like to achieve, and make clear in thought what it is and when you would like to achieve it.

Select a goal you would like to achieve, and establish clearly what it is and when you would like to achieve it (i.e. six months, twelve months, ten years).

Seated in a chair, get comfortable, and ensure arms and legs are uncrossed and your back is straight (loosen any tight clothing, belts, shoe etc). When you feel comfortable, close your eyes and begin focusing your attention on a comfortable breathing pattern. Then begin taking deep, full breaths. As you breathe in through your nose feel your abdomen expand. As you breathe out through your mouth feel your abdomen contract. Spend a few minutes consciously breathing deeply. Then allow yourself to breathe naturally. If you need to relax more fully, go through the 'relaxation' exercise before commencing your visualisation.

Meditation

Using your imagination, see yourself in the process of achieving your goal. What does it feel like? - bring your emotions into it - feel the joy and happiness. What are you wearing? What is in the room around you? See others supporting you and congratulating you. Make your visualisation as real as possible. Experience how empowered you feel - the courage, optimism and inner strength that you feel. Congratulate yourself!

Now see yourself further in the future - six months, one year, ten years - having achieved your goal. What is life like for you now that you have achieved your goal? Praise yourself for having the courage, determination and self-worth to follow through with your goals - for creating the life you want. Know within that you can pass through fears and achieve anything you want, now and in the future.

When your visualisation is complete, gently bring yourself back to waking consciousness.

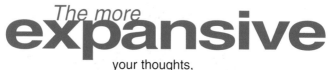

The more
expansive
your thoughts,
the more expansive the reality you create

Health:

This exercise may be used for general health and well-being, or a specific illness or disease.

Meditation

Seated in a chair, get comfortable, and ensure arms and legs are uncrossed and your back is straight (loosen any tight clothing, belts, shoes etc). When you feel comfortable, close your eyes and begin focusing your attention on a comfortable breathing pattern. Then begin taking deep, full breaths. As you breathe in through your nose feel your abdomen expand. As you breathe out through your mouth feel your abdomen contract. Spend a few minutes consciously breathing deeply. Then let go and allow yourself to breathe naturally. If you need to relax more fully, go through the 'relaxation' exercise before commencing your visualisation.

Imagine a beautiful white healing light shining and shimmering around you. As you breath in, visualise yourself inhaling this beautiful, healing light. See and feel it filling your body. Feel and see every cell vibrating in excellent health. Give your innate healing ability a form (a fairy, an animal, a wise sage, a light, a sound) - allow whatever comes. See this 'innate healer' working at its optimum - possessing vitality, energy, wisdom.

If you have an illness or area of disease, imagine your innate healer now healing this area in whatever way feels right. See the illness or area of disease dissolving, until all that is left are perfect cells vibrating and shimmering with light and perfect health.

When your visualisation is complete, gently bring yourself back to waking consciousness.

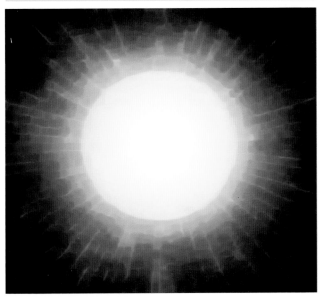

Self Acceptance and Self Love:

Seated in a chair, get comfortable, and ensure arms and legs are uncrossed and your back is straight (loosen any tight clothing, belts, shoes etc). When you feel comfortable, close your eyes and begin focusing your attention on a comfortable breathing pattern. Then begin taking deep, full breaths. As you breathe in through your nose feel your abdomen expand. As you breathe out through your mouth feel your abdomen contract. Spend a few minutes consciously breathing deeply. Then allow yourself to breathe naturally. If you need to relax more fully, go through the 'relaxation' exercise before commencing your visualisation.

Meditation

Visualise yourself as a small child. See yourself - beautiful; full of love and vitality; full of courage and optimism; enthusiasm and spontaneity. Go to your child and embrace it - it has been a long time since you've spent time together. Spend some time together - doing whatever it is that your child wants to do. Maybe your child would like to show you something. Maybe your child just wants to be cuddled. Allow whatever comes without judgement.

There are parts of your child that are wounded - does your child believe he/she isn't loved; isn't good enough; is unworthy? Does your child feel hurt and pain about something? In your visualisation go to your inner child as the adult you, and apologise for having neglected him/her. Let your child know that you never meant to hurt him/her with all your criticisms, and that you will be there for him/her in the future. Tell your child that he/she is loved; beautiful; worthy; talented; intelligent; courageous; helpful and useful. Tell your inner child that his/her expression brings great joy; that his/her creativity is celebrated; and his/her uniqueness is honoured by you. Acknowledge any sadness or hurt that your child has - do not criticise or judge - just understand and help to heal this inner child.

When your visualisation is complete, gently bring yourself back to waking consciousness.

Thoughts And Beliefs

The thoughts we choose to think create the experiences we have. Every conscious or unconscious thought we have, affects every feeling and every action we take.

Whatever we believe about something determines our attitude towards it; creates our feelings and directs our actions. **Belief, however, does not require that something be true. It only requires that we believe it to be true.** There is no area of our life in which we do not have a set of beliefs. If our beliefs are positive and nurturing, we are likely to have a positive experience of life. Whereas, if our beliefs are negative and limiting, we are likely to have a negative experience of life. **Most of our beliefs have become so habitual we rarely question them.** When we meditate and get in touch with our inner life of feelings, we begin to recognise our innermost core beliefs. Some of the beliefs may be nurturing, loving and nourishing and these should be celebrated. However, there may be many others which are damaging, unloving and limiting. As we discover and embrace core beliefs, we are able to heal, or alter them, if we truly desire it.

Our core beliefs profoundly affect our quality of life. For example, some common core beliefs may be: that it is hard to get by in the world; that we are not worthy; that we are not intelligent; that we are not allowed to express ourselves; that we are a failure; that we do not have enough time; that it is selfish to do things for ourselves; life is too hard; there are no opportunities. Most of us have many limiting thoughts and beliefs, both about who we are and about life.

Visualisation and affirmations are powerful tools for beginning to change and heal our limiting beliefs and patterns.

Affirmations

An affirmation is a strong, positive statement that something is already so. For example, if one of our core beliefs is "I never succeed" - we can start to replace it with a belief that we would rather have - "I always succeed". We affirm to ourselves the new positive belief. The practice of affirmation allows us to begin replacing our limiting and negative thoughts and beliefs with more positive beliefs.

Affirmations can be repeated silently, spoken aloud or written down. They can be incorporated into our meditations, or used in conjunction with our visualisations. They must be phrased in the present tense as if they already exist. Affirmations should always affirm what you want, not what you don't want, for example "I am healthy and strong" rather than "I am no longer sick".

An affirmation opens the way to change. The subconscious mind is very straightforward. It accepts whatever we tell it - it does not judge. Therefore, it is our choice as to whether we create positive beliefs that serve us; or simply react to negative, limiting beliefs that are old patterns.

Because many of us have limiting beliefs about our self-worth, it can help if we begin with basic affirmations that form the foundation for self-worth: "I am worthwhile"; "I love and approve of myself"; "I deserve ....."; "I am safe".

It is also powerful to state our intentions. Many of us get so caught up in the 'routine' of our lives, that we do not spend any time getting clear about what we want or desire out of life. To focus our energies, it is beneficial if we spend some time each week exploring and discovering what it is that would bring us happiness and make us feel alive.

Whatever these things are, we can focus our energies and call them to ourselves by affirming out loud what our intention is:

- I move beyond limiting beliefs and fears
- I experience radiant health and vitality
- I experience love and joy
- I experience abundance and prosperity.

Motivation And Dedication

In our busy lives it can be very easy to overlook making time for relaxation and meditation, because we have too much to do!

It can be a motivating force to remember that we will be more peaceful; have better concentration; think more clearly; be more creative; and have more energy following meditation. After meditating, we often get things done more effectively than if we didn't take the time to meditate.

Motivation And Dedication

The fact that we have made time for ourselves is also important. When taking time for ourselves and our well-being, we are affirming to ourselves that we are worth it - that we are deserving. This in turn has a positive effect on our self-worth and self-esteem.

Dedication and perseverance are central to the regular practice of meditation. At times we may be motivated by the insights, self-awareness and personal growth that is occurring. At other times, the process may begin to feel boring. It is at these times that our dedication and perseverance will be tested, and this is a natural experience for all of us. There may also be times when we experience states of inner turmoil, and want to turn away from the pain or challenges. The process of meditation does not unfold in a predictable manner, and for this reason it is better not to have expectations or judge our experiences.

If we find our meditations becoming 'lifeless' it may be time for a change. Do not be afraid to experiment and find out what gives new life to your meditations. To sustain interest in your journey try something different, such as:

- find a peaceful place in nature and reflect on your connectedness with mother earth
- use guided meditation/visualisation tapes or CD's for variation
- spend some time contemplating everything you feel grateful for and appreciate, and write them in a journal

- reflect on your own needs and desires in the following areas: family; relationships; work; spiritual and personal growth. Make notes in a journal of any thoughts or insights you may have
- contemplate an inspirational quotation such as "As man thinketh within himself, so he is", or reflect upon a poem. Make notes in a journal of any thoughts or insights you may have
- spend 15 minutes or so writing an affirmation many times, e.g. "I love and approve of myself" and notice the feelings, thoughts and body sensations that happen as you are writing it. Acknowledge these feelings and thoughts in your journal - they will lead you to the core beliefs you hold about yourself and life.

Participating in a meditation workshop will enliven creativity, and provide further ideas, tools and techniques. The group can also provide support, friendship, sharing and ideas for overcoming any challenges we may be experiencing. The dynamics are very powerful within group meditation - many people comment that they reach deeper meditative states in a group setting.

The primary motivation for our dedication and commitment to our journey will come from our ever-increasing experience of inner peace, happiness and the ability to meet life's challenges with clarity, courage and optimism.

Recommended Music For Meditation

O'Connor, Tony - Sea Australia

"Sea Australia is a selection of tracks from several of Tony O'Connor's multi-award winning albums, each piece a musical masterpiece inspired by the ocean and the coastlines of this wonderful country. Relax to the waves crashing, whales calling and gentle music by Australia's most popular creator of Music for Relaxation".

Oldfield, Terry - Resonance

"If the most heavenly of noble emotions could find voice, it would be that of the haunting Pan Pipes. Alluring, mysterious and compelling, the lingering quality of this music draws the listener right to the heart-beat of the Earth .... An unexcelled performance of passionate calm"

Stagg, Hilary - The Edge Of Forever

"Harpist Hilary Stagg has created a masterpiece with The Edge of Forever. Once again, through the captivating sound of his harp combined with flute and keyboards, Hilary takes you to a musical sanctuary where serenity, power and tranquillity all await"

Thornton, Phil - Initiation

"Initiation weaves the haunting voice of whales and birds into the strong, mellow Dreamworld of the Didgeridoo. From the fascinating and earthy sounds of this most basic of natural instruments to the superb complexity of modern keyboards, we are enmeshed in a world of compelling imagination ..."

Wheater, Tim - A Calmer Panorama

"Exquisitely beautiful flutes that continuously ebb and flow, blending harmoniously with the natural music of falling water and calling birds; evoking dreamy images of shafted sunlight on sparkling waters"

Recommended Further Reading

Gawain, Shakti - Creative Visualisation
"This metaphysical book contains meditations, exercises and techniques to assist us in increasing our personal mastery of life"

Gawler, Ian - Meditation Pure & Simple
"In this book, Ian Gawler distills the heart and essence of meditation practice and presents techniques for relaxation and meditation"

Wilson, Paul - Instant Calm
"This book clearly describes over a hundred calming techniques for well-being based on meditation, acupressure, self-hypnosis, psychotherapy, aromatherapy, exercise and diet"

Recommended Guided Meditations/Visualisations

Everard, Margaret - Ocean Blue
"Guided journeys of deep relaxation and meditation which allow you to release stress and learn to be in harmony with yourself. Follow the path as it leads to sand, sea and dolphins. Visit the rainforest and the waterfall at its heart. Experience the healing pool and its tranquil waters. Return from these journeys calm, energised and in touch"

James, Chris - Harmonic Meditation
"The guided relaxation ... is wonderful for stress reduction. Chris helps you to relax your body and your mind and then uses his ability to sing vocal overtones (singing two pure notes at once) to relax and align the energy of your body..."

Linn, Denise - Cellular Regeneration - How To Heal
"This tape series combines Denise's extensive knowledge and personal experience to assist others in their search for healing, self-improvement and empowerment. Discover profound healing and transformation as a result of listening to these very powerful tapes"

Pinkerton, Margaret - Moving On
"... Use this tape when you wish to relax and experience tranquillity, let go of burdens, heal the emptiness within, deal with life's obstacles, accept yourself and others, discover the real nature of your soul"

*The Journey of a Thousand Miles Begins with
a First Step...*

the
First Steps
series

- First Steps to Meditation
- First Steps to Massage
- First Steps to Chi Kung
- First Steps to Tarot
- First Steps to Dream Power
- First Steps to Yoga

Further titles following shortly:

- First Steps to Reflexology
- First Steps to Feng Shui
- First Steps to Managing Stress
- First Steps to Astrology
- First Steps to Chinese Herbal Medicine
- First Steps to Acupressure

First Steps to...

•AXIOM PUBLISHING
Unit 2, 1 Union Street, Stepney, South Australia, 5069